C000218286

Air Fryer Poultry Cooking Guide

A Beginner's guide to Simple and Delicious Poultry Dishes for Air Fryer

By Donna Thomson

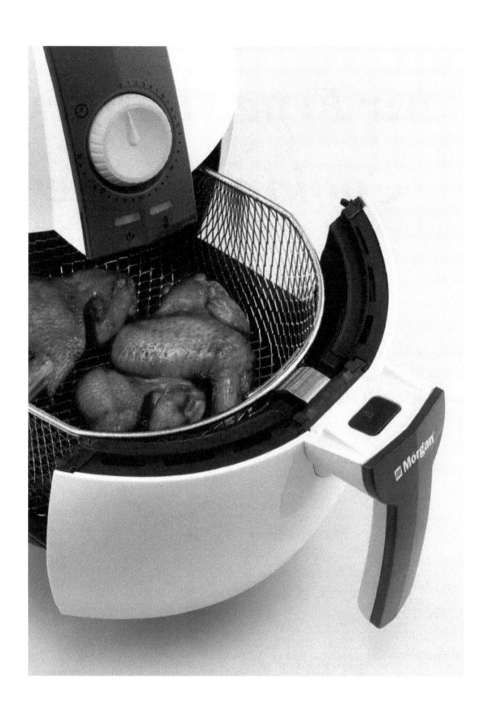

© Copyright 2021 - All rights reserved.

The content contained within this book may not be reproduced, duplicated or transmitted without direct written permission from the author or the publisher.

Under no circumstances will any blame or legal responsibility be held against the publisher, or author, for any damages, reparation, or monetary loss due to the information contained within this book. Either directly or indirectly.

Legal Notice:

This book is copyright protected. This book is only for personal use. You cannot amend, distribute, sell, use, quote or paraphrase any part, or the content within this book, without the consent of the author or publisher.

Disclaimer Notice:

Please note the information contained within this document is for educational and entertainment purposes only. All effort has been executed to present accurate, up to date, and reliable, complete information. No warranties of any kind are declared or implied. Readers acknowledge that the author is not engaging in the rendering of legal, financial, medical or professional advice.

The content within this book has been derived from various sources. Please consult a licensed professional before attempting any techniques outlined in this book.

By reading this document, the reader agrees that under no circumstances is the author responsible for any losses, direct or indirect, which are incurred as a result of the use of information contained within this document, including, but not limited to, — errors, omissions, or inaccuracies.

Table of Contents

Chicken BBQ Recipe from Italy 9

Chicken BBQ Recipe from Peru 11

Chicken BBQ with Sweet 'n Sour Sauce 13

Chicken Fry Recipe in the Mediterranean 15

Chicken Grill Recipe from California 18

Chicken in Packets Southwest Style 20

Chicken Kebab with Aleppo 'n Yogurt 22

Chicken Meatballs with Miso-Ginger 24

Chicken Pot Pie with Coconut Milk 26

Chicken Roast with Pineapple Salsa 29

Chicken Strips with Garlic, Onion 'n Paprika Blend 31

Chicken Tikka Masala Kebab 33

Chicken with Ginger-Cilantro Coconut Milk Marinade 36

Chicken with Peach Glaze 38

Chicken-Parm, Broccoli 'n Mushroom Bake 40

Chicken-Penne Pesto 42

Chicken-Veggie Fusilli Casserole 45

Chili, Lime & Corn Chicken BBQ 47

Chinese Five Spiced Marinated Chicken 49

Chipotle Chicken ala King 51

Chipotle-Garlic Smoked Wings 54

Chives, Eggs 'n Ham Casserole...56

Chorizo-Oregano Frittata..58

Cilantro-Lime 'n Liquid Smoke Chicken Grill...........................60

Coco Milk 'n Paprika-Oregano Marinated Drumsticks 62

Copycat KFC Chicken Strips 64

Creamy Chicken 'n Pasta Tetrazzini......................................67

Creamy Chicken 'n Rice 69

Creamy Chicken Breasts with crumbled Bacon 71

Creamy Chicken-Veggie Pasta 73

Creamy Coconut Egg 'n Mushroom Bake 76

Creamy Scrambled Eggs with Broccoli...................................78

Creamy Turkey Bake 80

Crispy 'n Salted Chicken Meatballs.......................................82

Crispy Fried Buffalo Chicken Breasts 84

Crispy Tender Parmesan Chicken 86

Curried Rice 'n Chicken Bake 88

Curry-Peanut Butter Rubbed Chicken 90

Dijon-Garlic Thighs..92

Drunken Chicken Jerk Spiced..93

Easy Chicken Fried Rice 95

Easy Fried Chicken Southern Style...97

Easy How-To Hard Boil Egg in Air Fryer 98

Eggs 'n Turkey Bake 100

Eggs Benedict on English Muffins..102

Eggs, Cauliflower 'n Broccoli Brekky....................................104

French Toast with Apples 'n Raisins 106

Garam Masala 'n Yogurt Marinated Chicken 109

Chicken BBQ Recipe from Italy

Servings per Recipe: 2

Cooking Time: 40 minutes

Ingredients

- 1 tablespoon fresh Italian parsley /15G
- 1 tablespoon minced garlic /15G
- 1-pound boneless chicken breasts /450G
- 2 tablespoons tomato paste /30ML
- Salt and pepper to taste

Instructions:

1) Add all ingredients except for the corn in a Ziploc bag. Allow to marinate inside the fridge for a couple of hours.
2) Preheat the air fryer to 390° F or 199°C .
3) Place the grill pan accessory inside the air fryer.
4) Grill the chicken for 40 minutes.

Nutrition information:

- Calories per serving: 292
- Carbs: 6.6g
- Protein: 52.6g
- Fat: 6.1g

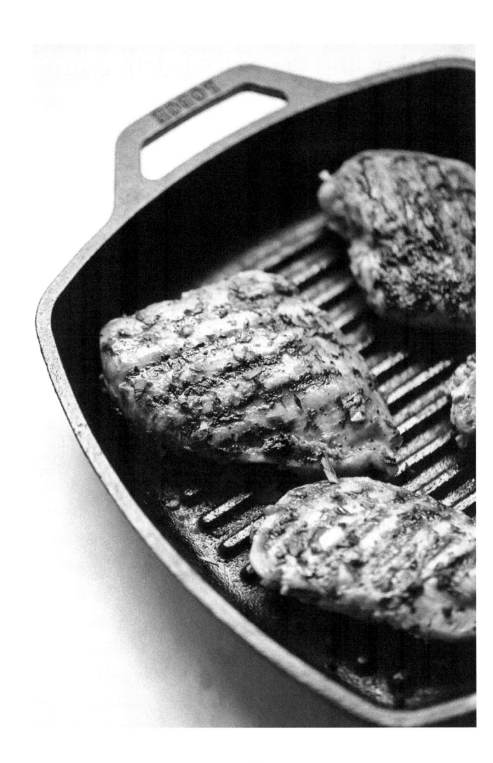

Chicken BBQ Recipe from Peru

Servings per Recipe: 4

Cooking Time: 40 minutes

Ingredients:

- ½ teaspoon dried oregano /2.5G
- 1 teaspoon paprika /5G
- 1/3 cup soy sauce /83ML
- 2 ½ pounds chicken, quartered /1125G
- 2 tablespoons fresh lime juice /30ML
- 2 teaspoons ground cumin /10G
- 5 cloves of garlic, minced

Instructions:

1) Add all ingredients in a Ziploc bag and shake to combine everything.
2) Place in a fridge and allow to marinate for few hours.
3) Preheat mid-air fryer to 390° F or 199°C .
4) Place the grill pan accessory inside the air fryer.
5) Grill the chicken for 40 minutes. Flip the chicken every 10 minutes for even grilling.

Nutrition information:

- Calories per serving: 377
- Carbs: 7.9g

- Protein: 59.7g
- Fat: 11.8g

Chicken BBQ with Sweet 'n Sour Sauce

Servings per Recipe: 6

Cooking Time: 40 minutes

Ingredients:

- ¼ cup minced garlic /32.5G
- ¼ cup tomato paste /32.5G
- ¾ cup minced onion /98G
- ¾ cup sugar 98G
- 1 cup soy sauce /250ML
- 1 cup water 250ML
- 1 cup white vinegar 250ML
- 6 chicken drumsticks
- Salt and pepper to taste

Instructions:

1) Place all Ingredients in the Ziploc bag
2) Place the Ziploc bag in a fridge and allow to marinate for 120 minutes.
3) Preheat the air fryer to 390° F or 199°C .
4) Place the grill pan accessory in the air fryer.
5) Grill the chicken for 40 minutes.
6) Flip the chicken every 10 minutes for only grilling.
7) Meanwhile, pour the marinade in a saucepan, place on a medium-flame and allow to warm till the sauce thickens.

8) Brush the chicken lavishly with sauce. Serve and enjoy.

Nutrition information:

- Calories per serving: 407
- Carbs:29.6 g
- Protein: 27.8g
- Fat: 19.7g

Chicken Fry Recipe in the Mediterranean

Servings per Recipe: 2

Cooking Time: 21 minutes

Ingredients:

- 2 boneless skinless chicken white meat halves (6 ounces or 180G each)
- 3 tablespoons organic olive oil /45ML
- 6 pitted Greek or ripe olives, sliced
- 2 tablespoons capers, drained /30G
- 1/2-pint grape tomatoes
- 1/4 teaspoon salt /1.25G
- 1/4 teaspoon pepper /1.25G

Instructions:

1) Grease a pan lightly with oil.

2) Add chicken and season with pepper and salt to taste.

3) Preheat air fryer at 390O F or 199°C . Place chicken in the air fryer, allow each side to Brown for 3 minutes.

4) Add capers, olives, tomatoes, and oil. Mix well.

5) Cook for 15 minutes, cook at 330O F or 166°C .

6) Serve and enjoy

Nutrition Information:

- Calories per Serving: 330
- Carbs: 6.0g
- Protein: 36.0g
- Fat: 18.0g

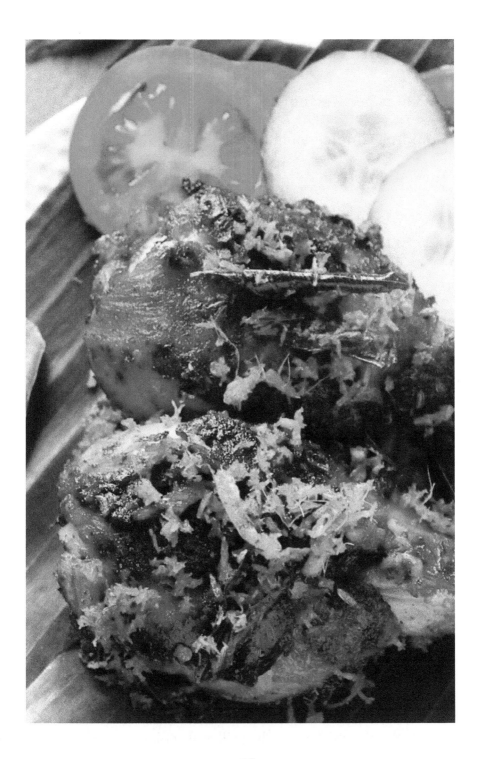

Chicken Grill Recipe from California

Servings per Recipe: 4

Cooking Time: 40 minutes

Ingredients:

- ¾ cup balsamic vinegar /188ML
- 1 teaspoon garlic powder /5G
- 2 tablespoons extra virgin organic olive oil /30ML
- 2 tablespoons honey /30ML
- 2 teaspoons Italian seasoning /10G
- 4 boneless chicken breasts
- 4 slices mozzarella
- 4 slices of avocado
- 4 slices of tomato
- Balsamic vinegar for drizzling
- Salt and pepper to taste

Instructions:

1) Mix the balsamic vinegar, garlic powder, honey, organic olive oil, Italian seasoning, salt, pepper, and chicken in a Ziploc bag. Allow to marinate in the fridge for about 2 hours.
2) Preheat air fryer to 390° F or 199°C .
3) Place the grill pan accessory in the air fryer.
4) Put the chicken on the grill and cook for 40 minutes.

5) Flip the chicken every 10 Minutes to grill evenly.

6) Serve the chicken with mozzarella, avocado, and tomato. Drizzle with balsamic vinegar.

Nutrition information:

- Calories per serving: 853
- Carbs: 43.2g
- Protein:69.4 g
- Fat: 44.7g

Chicken in Packets Southwest Style

Servings per Recipe: 4

Cooking Time: 40 minutes

Ingredients:

- 1 can black beans, rinsed and drained
- 1 cup cilantro, chopped /130G
- 1 cup commercial salsa /130G
- 1 cup corn kernels, frozen /130G
- 1 cup Mexican cheese blend, shredded /130G
- 4 chicken breasts
- 4 lime wedges
- 4 teaspoons taco seasoning /20G
- Salt and pepper to taste

Instructions:

1) Preheat air fryer to 390° F or 199°C.
2) Place the grill pan accessory in the air fryer.
3) Place the chicken breasts on a large aluminium foil, and season with salt and pepper to taste.
4) Add the corn, commercial salsa beans, and taco seasoning.
5) Wrap the foil and crumple the sides.
6) Place on the grill pan and cook for 40 minutes.
7) Before serving, top with cheese, cilantro and lime wedges.

Nutrition information:

- Calories per serving: 837
- Carbs: 47.5g
- Protein: 80.1g
- Fat: 36.2g

Chicken Kebab with Aleppo 'n Yogurt

Servings per Recipe: 2

Cooking Time: 20 minutes

Ingredients:

- 1 tablespoon Aleppo pepper /15G

- 1 tablespoon extra-virgin olive oil /15ML
- 1 tablespoon red wine vinegar /15ML
- 1 tablespoon tomato paste /15ML
- 1 teaspoon coarse kosher salt /5G
- 1 teaspoon freshly ground black pepper /5G
- 3 garlic cloves, peeled, flattened
- 1-pound skinless boneless chicken (thighs and/or breast halves), cut into 1 1/4-inch cube /450G
- 1 unpeeled lemon; 1/2 thinly sliced into rounds, 1/2 cut into wedges for serving
- 1/3 cup plain whole-milk Greek-style yogurt /88ML

Instructions:

1) Add all ingredients to a bowl and mix properly. Place in a fridge and allow to marinate for nothing short of an hour.
2) Skewer chicken and place in the air fryer skewer rack.
3) For 10 minutes, cook at 360° F or 183°C . Turnover skewers after 5 minutes of cooking.
4) Serve with lemon wedges and enjoy.

Nutrition Information:

- Calories per Serving: 336
- Carbs: 7.0g
- Protein: 53.6g
- Fat: 10.4g

Chicken Meatballs with Miso-Ginger

Servings per Recipe: 4

Cooking Time: 10 Minutes

Ingredients:

- 1 1/2 teaspoons white miso paste /7.5ML
- 1 large egg
- 1 teaspoon finely grated ginger /5G
- 1/4 cup panko (Japanese breadcrumbs), or fresh breadcrumbs /32.5 g
- 1/4 teaspoon kosher salt /1.25G
- 2 tablespoons sliced scallions /30G
- 2 teaspoons low-sodium soy sauce /10ML
- 3/4-pound ground chicken /338G

Instructions:

1) Add soy sauce, miso paste, and ginger to a medium-sized bowl. Mix all ingredients. Set aside.
2) Add ground chicken, large egg, scallions, and salt to another bowl and mix well with hands. Add panko and half of the sauce. Mix well continuously.
3) Evenly form 12 balls with the mix. Thread into 4 skewers.
4) Place on skewer rack.

5) Cook for 2 minutes at 390° F or 199°C . Baste with remaining sauce, turnover and cook for another 2 minutes. Baste with sauce again and cook for another 2 minutes.

6) Serve and enjoy.

Nutrition Information:

- Calories per Serving: 145
- Carbs: 4.2g
- Protein: 17.4g
- Fat: 8.2g

Chicken Pot Pie with Coconut Milk

Serves: 8

Cooking Time: 30 Minutes

Ingredients:

- ¼ small onion, chopped
- ½ cup broccoli, chopped/65G
- ¾ cup coconut milk /188ML
- 1 cup chicken broth /250ML
- 1/3 cup coconut flour /43G
- 1-pound ground chicken /450G
- 2 cloves of garlic, minced
- 2 tablespoons butter /30G
- 4 ½ tablespoons butter, melted 75ML
- 4 eggs
- Salt and pepper to taste

Instructions:

1) Preheat the air fryer for 5 minutes.
2) Place 2 tablespoons of butter, broccoli, onion, garlic, coconut milk, chicken broth, and ground chicken inside a baking dish. Mix well. Season with salt and pepper to taste.
3) Add the butter, coconut flour, and eggs into a mixing bowl. Mix well.

4) Sprinkle the top of the chicken and broccoli mixture with the coconut flour dough.

5) Place the dish inside the air fryer.

6) Cook for 30 minutes at 325° F or 163°C .

Nutrition information:

- Calories per serving: 366
- Carbohydrates: 3.4g
- Protein: 21.8g
- Fat: 29.5g

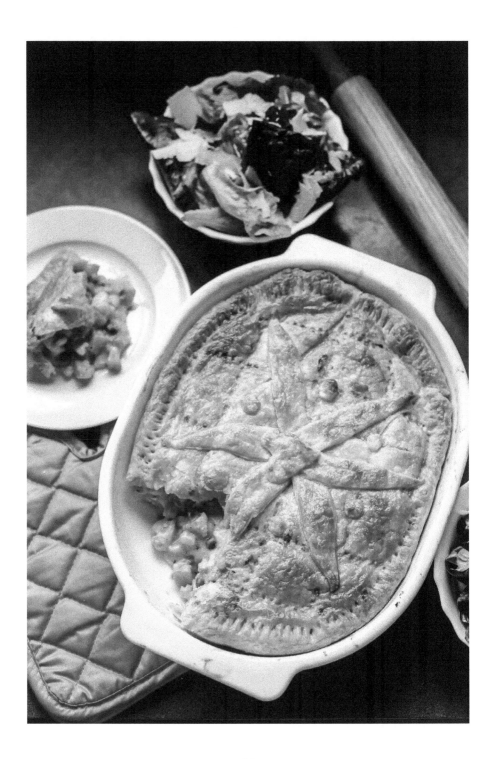

Chicken Roast with Pineapple Salsa

Servings per Recipe: 2

Cooking Time: 45 minutes

Ingredients:

- ¼ cup extra virgin organic olive oil /62.5ML
- ¼ cup freshly chopped cilantro /32.5G
- 1 avocado, diced
- 1-pound boneless chicken breasts /450G
- 2 cups canned pineapples /260G
- 2 teaspoons honey /10ML
- Juice from 1 lime
- Salt and pepper to taste

Instructions:

1) Preheat the air fryer to 390° F or 199°C .
2) Place the grill pan accessory in the air fryer.
3) Place chicken breast in a bowl. Season with lime juice, organic olive oil, honey, salt, and pepper.
4) Place on the grill pan and cook for 45 minutes.
5) Flip the chicken every 10 minutes for even grilling.
6) Once the chicken is cooked, serve with pineapples, cilantro, and avocado.

Nutrition information:

- Calories per serving: 744
- Carbs: 57.4g
- Protein: 54.7g
- Fat: 32.8g

Chicken Strips with Garlic, Onion 'n Paprika Blend

Serves: 4

Cooking Time: 25 minutes

Ingredients:

- ¼ cup vegetable oil /62.5ML
- 1 cup coconut milk /250ML
- 1 tablespoon cayenne /15G
- 1 teaspoon garlic powder /5G
- 1 teaspoon onion powder /5G
- 1-pound chicken breast, cut into strips /450G
- 2 cups almond flour /260G
- 2 eggs
- 2 tablespoons paprika /30G
- Salt and pepper to taste

Instructions:

1) Place chicken meat in a bowl. Season with salt and pepper to taste. Set aside.
2) In a mixing bowl, combine the eggs and coconut milk. Set aside.
3) In another bowl, mix the almond flour, paprika, garlic powder, and onion powder.

4) Soak the chicken meat within the egg mixture then dredge within the flour mixture.

5) Place in the air fryer basket.

6) Cook for 25 minutes at 350° F or 177°C.

7) Meanwhile, prepare the new sauce by combining the red pepper cayenne and vegetable.

8) Sprinkle over chicken once cooked.

Nutrition information:

- Calories per serving: 539.7
- Carbohydrates: 8.6g
- Protein: 29.8g
- Fat: 42.9g

Chicken Tikka Masala Kebab

Servings per Recipe: 4

Cooking Time: 20 Minutes

Ingredients:

1 boneless, skinless chicken white meat, cut into bite-sized pieces

- 1 cup thick yogurt /250ML
- 1 medium bell pepper, cut into bite-sized pieces
- 1 tbsp fresh ginger paste /15G
- 1 tsp Garam masala /5G
- 1 tsp turmeric powder /5G
- 2 tbsp coriander powder /30G
- 2 tbsp cumin powder /30G
- 2 tbsp red chili powder /30G
- 2 tsp olive oil /10ML
- 8 cherry tomatoes
- Salt to taste

Instructions:

1) Add all ingredients except for chicken, bell pepper, and tomatoes in a bowl. Mix well. Add chicken, mix, place in a fridge and marinate for about an hour.

2) Skewer chicken, bell pepper, chicken, cherry tomato, chicken, then tomato and pepper. Repeat for remaining skewers.

3) Place skewer in skewer rack, for 10 minutes, cook on 390° F or 199°C. After 5 minutes turnover skewer to cook evenly.

4) Serve and enjoy.

Nutrition Information:

- Calories per Serving: 273
- Carbs: 17.4g
- Protein: 20.3g
- Fat: 13.5g

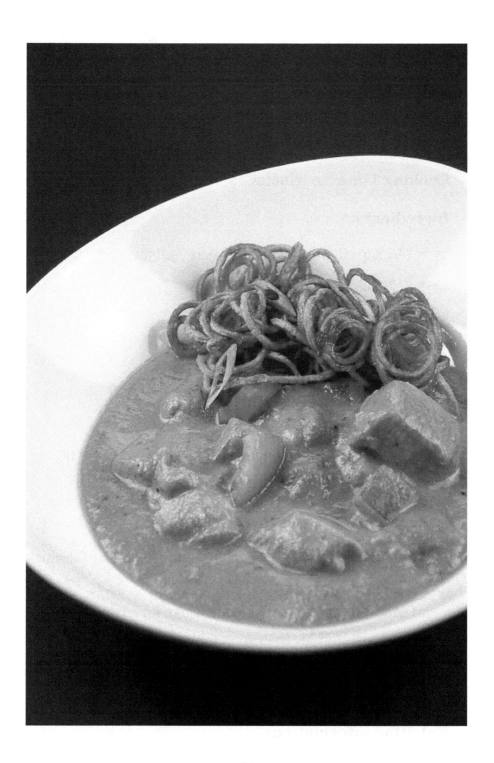

Chicken with Ginger-Cilantro Coconut Milk Marinade

Serves: 5

Cooking Time: 20 minutes

Ingredients:

- ¼ cup cilantro leaves, chopped /32.5G
- ½ cup coconut milk /125ML
- 1 tablespoon grated ginger /15G
- 1 tablespoon minced garlic /15G
- 1 teaspoon garam masala /5G
- 1 teaspoon smoked paprika /5G
- 1 teaspoon turmeric /5G
- 1-pound chicken tenders, cut by 50 per cent /450G
- Salt and pepper to taste

Instructions

1) Place all ingredients in a bowl and stir to coat the chicken tenders.
2) Allow to marinate inside the fridge for a couple of hours.
3) Preheat mid-air fryer for 5 minutes.
4) Place the chicken pieces in the air fryer basket.
5) Cook for 20 minutes at 400° F or 205°C .

Nutrition information:

- Calories per serving: 1198
- Carbohydrates: 19.5g
- Protein: 15.8g
- Fat: 117.4

Chicken with Peach Glaze

Servings per Recipe: 4

Cooking Time: 40 minutes

Ingredients:

- 1 jalapeno chopped
- 1 tablespoon chili powder /15G
- 1 tablespoon minced garlic /15G
- 1 tablespoons Dijon mustard /15G
- 2 cups peach preserves /260G
- 2 pounds chicken thighs /900G
- 2 tablespoons soy sauce /30ML
- 3 tablespoons olive oil /45ML
- Salt and pepper to taste

Instructions:

1) Place all ingredients inside a Ziploc bag and allow to set in the fridge for 2 hours.
2) Preheat the air fryer to 390° F or 199°C .
3) Place the grill pan accessory in the air fryer.
4) Grill for 40 minutes while turning over the chicken every 10 minutes.
5) Meanwhile, pour the marinade in a saucepan and allow to simmer for 5 minutes until the sauce thickens.
6) Brush the chicken with the sauce before serving.

Nutrition information:

- Calories per serving: 730
- Carbs: 31.7g
- Protein: 39.4g
- Fat: 49.5g

Chicken-Parm, Broccoli 'n Mushroom Bake

Servings per Recipe: 2

Cooking Time: 40 minutes

Ingredients:

- 1 (13.5 ounces) can spinach, drained /405G
- 1 cup shredded mozzarella cheese /130G
- 1/2 (10.75 ounces) can condensed cream of mushroom soup /322.5ML
- 1/3 cup bacon bits /43G
- 1/4 cup grated Parmesan cheese /32.5G
- 1/4 cup half-and-half /32.5G
- 1-1/2 teaspoons Italian seasoning /7.5G
- 1-1/2 teaspoons freshly squeezed lemon juice /7.5ML
- 1-1/2 teaspoons minced garlic /7.5ML
- 2 ounces fresh mushrooms, sliced /60G
- 2 skinless, boneless chicken halves
- 2 tablespoons butter /30G

Instructions:

1) Lightly grease the baking pan. Add chicken breast, cook for 20 minutes at 360° F or 183°C . Turnover the chicken breast after 10 minutes of cooking. After which you can transfer it to a plate and set it aside.

2) In the same baking pan, melt butter. Stir in Parmesan cheese, half and half, Italian seasoning, mushroom soup, fresh lemon juice, and garlic. Mix well and cook for 5 minutes or until well cooked.

3) Stir in spinach and chicken. Top with bacon bits and mozzarella cheese.

4) Cook for 15 minutes at 390° F or 199°C until tops are lightly browned.

5) Serve and enjoy.

Nutrition Information:

- Calories per Serving: 659
- Carbs: 17.6g
- Protein: 61.6g
- Fat: 38.0g

Chicken-Penne Pesto

Servings per Recipe: 3

Cooking Time: 25 minutes

Ingredients:

- 1 cup shredded Italian cheese blend /130G
- 1/3 cup milk /83ML
- 1/4 (15 ounces) can crushed tomatoes /450G
- 1/4 (15 ounces) jar Alfredo sauce /450ML
- 1/4 (15 ounces) jar pesto sauce /450ML
- 1-1/2 cups cubed cooked chicken /195G
- 2 tablespoons grated Parmesan cheese /30G
- 2 tablespoons seasoned bread crumbs /30G
- 3/4 cup fresh baby spinach /97
- 3/4 teaspoon organic olive oil /3.75ML
- 4-ounce penne pasta, cooked based on manufacturer's Instructions /120G

Instructions:

1) Add essential olive oil, Parmesan, and bread crumbs to a bowl. Mix well and Set aside.

2) Lightly grease the baking pan of the air fryer. While mixing add milk, pesto sauce, alfredo sauce, tomatoes, spinach, and Italian cheese blend. Mix well. Add in cooked pasta and mix well to coat. Sprinkle bread crumb mixture evenly on top.

3) Cook at 360° F or 183°C for 25 minutes until tops are lightly browned.

4) Serve and enjoy.

Nutrition Information:

- Calories per Serving: 729
- Carbs: 40.7g
- Protein: 45.4g
- Fat: 47.2g

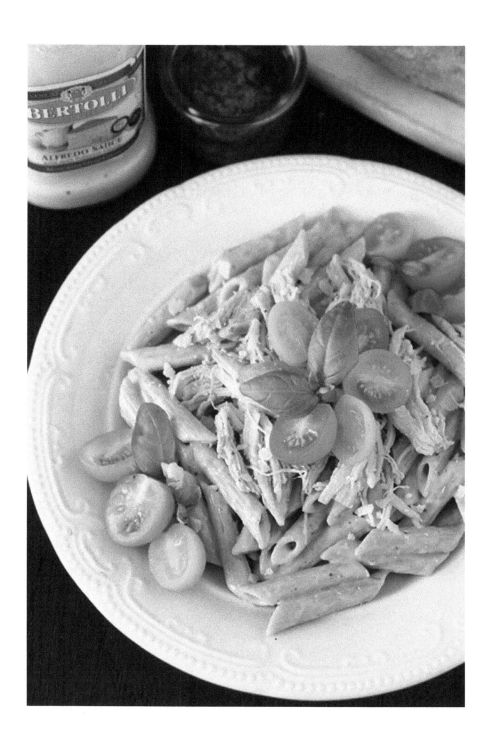

Chicken-Veggie Fusilli Casserole

Servings per Recipe: 3

Cooking Time: 30 Minutes

Ingredients:

- 1 cup frozen mixed vegetables /130G
- 1 tablespoon butter, melted /15ML
- 1 tablespoon grated Parmesan cheese /15G
- 1 tablespoon olive oil /15ML
- 1/2 (10.75 ounces) can condensed cream of chicken soup /322.5ML
- 1/2 (10.75 ounces) can condensed cream of mushroom soup /322.5ML
- 1/2 cup dry bread crumbs /65G
- 1/2 cup dry fusilli pasta, cooked based on manufacturer's instructions /65G
- 1-1/2 teaspoons dried basil /7.5G
- 1-1/2 teaspoons dried minced onion /7.5G
- 1-1/2 teaspoons dried parsley /7.5G
- 3 chicken tenderloins, cut into chunks
- garlic powder to taste
- salt and pepper to taste

Instructions:

1) Grease baking pan of air fryer lightly with olive oil. Add chicken. Season with parsley, basil, garlic powder, pepper, salt, and minced onion.

2) Cook at 360° F or 183°C for 10 minutes. After 5 minutes stir the chicken to ensure even cooking.

3) Remove the basket, stir in mixed vegetables, cream of mushroom soup, cream of chicken soup, and cooked pasta. Mix well.

4) Mix melted butter, parmesan, and bread crumbs in a bowl. Evenly spread on the top of casserole.

5) Cook for 20 minutes at 390° F or 199°C .

6) Serve and enjoy.

Nutrition Information:

- Calories per Serving: 399
- Carbs: 35.4g
- Protein: 19.8g
- Fat: 19.8g

Chili, Lime & Corn Chicken BBQ

Servings per Recipe: 4

Cooking Time: 40 minutes

Ingredients:

- ½ teaspoon cumin /2.5G
- 1 tablespoon lime juice /15ML
- 1 teaspoon chili powder /5G
- 2 chicken breasts
- 2 chicken thighs
- 2 cups barbecue sauce /500ML
- 2 teaspoons grated lime zest /10G
- 4 ears of corn, cleaned
- Salt and pepper to taste

Instructions:

1) Place all ingredients inside a Ziploc bag except for the corn. Allow to marinate in the fridge for a couple of hours.
2) Preheat mid-air fryer to 390° F or 199°C .
3) Place the grill pan accessory inside the air fryer.
4) Grill the chicken and corn for 40 minutes.
5) Meanwhile, pour the marinade inside a saucepan over medium heat until it thickens.

6) Before serving, brush the chicken and corn with the sauce.

Nutrition information:

- Calories per serving: 849
- Carbs: 87.7g
- Protein: 52.3g
- Fat: 32.1g

Chinese Five Spiced Marinated Chicken

Servings per Recipe: 4

Cooking Time: 40 minutes

Ingredients

- ¼ cup hoisin sauce /62.5ML
- 1 ¼ teaspoons sesame oil /6.25ML
- 1 ½ teaspoon five-spice powder /7.5G
- 2 chicken breasts, halved
- 2 tablespoons rice vinegar /30ML
- 2 teaspoons brown sugar /10G
- 3 ½ teaspoons grated ginger /17.5G
- 3 ½ teaspoons honey /17.5ML
- 3 cucumbers, sliced
- Salt and pepper to taste

Instructions:

1) Place all ingredients except the cucumber inside a Ziploc bag.
2) Allow to marinate in the fridge for a couple of hours.
3) Preheat air fryer to 390° F or 199°C .
4) Place the grill pan accessory within the air fryer.
5) Grill for 40 minutes and turn over the chicken frequently.
6) Serve chicken with cucumber once cooked.

Nutrition information:

- Calories per serving: 330
- Carbs:16.7 g
- Protein: 31.2g
- Fat: 15.4g

Chipotle Chicken ala King

Servings per Recipe: 4

Cooking Time: 40 minutes

Ingredients:

- 1 tablespoon sour cream /15ML
- 1 teaspoon ground cumin /5G
- 4 corn tortillas, cut into quarters
- 1/2 (10.75 ounces) can condensed cream of mushroom soup /322.5G
- 1/2 (10.75 ounces) can condensed cream of chicken soup /322.5G
- 1-1/2 teaspoons vegetable oil /7.5ML
- 1/2 white onion, diced
- 1/2 red bell pepper, diced
- 1/2 green bell pepper, diced
- 1/2 (10 ounces) can diced tomatoes with green chile peppers (including RO*TEL®) /300G
- 1/2 cup chicken broth /125ML
- 1/2 teaspoon ancho chile powder /2.5G
- 1/2 cooked chicken, torn into shreds or cut into chunks
- 1/4 teaspoon dried oregano /1.25G
- 1/4-pound shredded Cheddar cheese /1.25G
- 1/8 teaspoon chipotle chile powder /0.625G

Instructions:

1) Use vegetable oil to lightly grease the baking pan of the air fryer. Add bell pepper, red bell pepper, and onion. For 5 minutes, cook at 360° F or 183°C .

2) Add chipotle chile powder, oregano, ancho chile powder, cumin, sour cream, chicken broth, diced tomatoes, cream of chicken soup, and cream of mushroom soup in a large bowl and mix well.

3) Pour cooked sweet pepper into the bowl of sauce and mix well.

4) Add a few scoops of sauce to the bottom of the air fryer baking pan. Place ½ of chicken on top of the sauce, also top with 1/3 cheese, cover using a layer of corn tortilla. Repeat the process until all ingredients are used up.

5) Cover the pan with foil.

6) Cook for 25 minutes. Uncover and continue cooking for an additional 10 Minutes.

7) Serve and enjoy.

Nutrition Information:

- Calories per Serving: 482
- Carbs: 25.1g
- Protein: 32.1g
- Fat: 28.1g

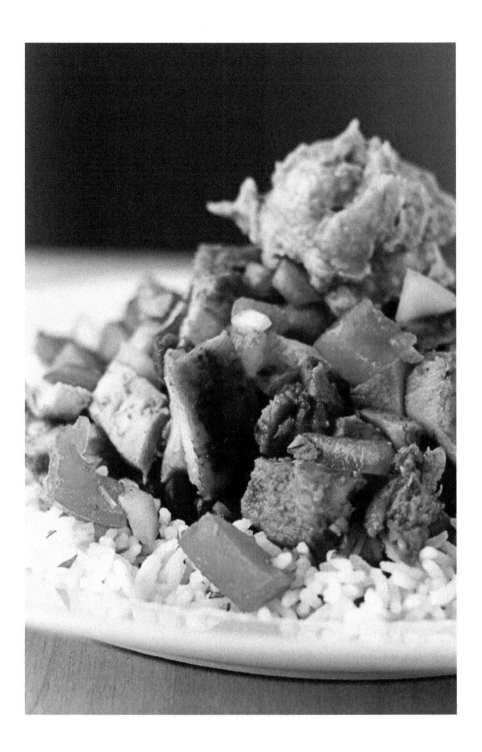

Chipotle-Garlic Smoked Wings

Servings per Recipe: 8

Cooking Time: 30 minutes

Ingredients:

- ½ cup barbecue sauce /125ML
- 1 tablespoon chili powder /15G
- 1 tablespoon garlic powder /15G
- 1 tablespoon liquid smoke seasoning /15G
- 1 teaspoon chipotle chili powder /5G
- 1 teaspoon mustard powder /5G
- 3 tablespoons paprika /45G
- 4 pounds chicken wings /1800G
- 4 teaspoons salt /20G

Instructions:

1) Place all ingredients in the Ziploc bag. Shake vigorously.
2) Allow to marinate for a couple of hours inside the fridge.
3) Preheat the air fryer to 390° F or 199°C .
4) Place the grill pan accessory within the air fryer.
5) Grill the chicken for 30 minutes.
6) Flip the chicken every 10 minutes.
7) Meanwhile, pour the marinade in the saucepan and heat over medium flame until the sauce thickens.
8) Brush the chicken with the sauce.

Nutrition information:

- Calories per serving: 324
- Carbs: 10.8g
- Protein: 50.7g
- Fat: 8.6g

Chives, Eggs 'n Ham Casserole

Serves: 4

Cooking Time: 15

Ingredients:

- 1 egg, whole
- 2 tablespoons butter, unsalted /30G
- 2 tablespoons coconut cream /30ML
- 2 teaspoon fresh chives, chopped /10
- 3 uncured ham, chopped
- 4 large eggs, beaten
- Salt and pepper to taste

Instructions:

1) Preheat the air fryer for 5 minutes.
2) Add the beaten eggs, coconut cream, butter, and chives to a bowl. Season with salt and pepper to taste.
3) Pour in a baking dish and sprinkle ham on top.
4) Crack 1 egg at the top.
5) Place in the air fryer.
6) Cook for 15 minutes at 350° F or 177°C .

Nutrition information:

- Calories per serving: 178
- Carbohydrates: 2.6g

- Protein: 6.4g
- Fat: 15.8g

Chorizo-Oregano Frittata

Serves: 6

Cooking Time: 15

Ingredients:

- ½ chorizo sausage, sliced
- ½ zucchini, sliced
- 3 large eggs, beaten
- 3 tablespoons organic olive oil /45ML
- A dash of oregano
- A dash of Spanish paprika

Instructions:

1) Preheat the air fryer for 5 minutes.
2) Add all ingredients to a mixing bowl and mix properly.
3) Pour the mixture into an already greased baking dish that will fit inside the air fryer.
4) Place the baking dish inside the air fryer.
5) Close and cook for 15 minutes at 350° F or 177°C .

Nutrition information:

- Calories per serving: 94
- Carbohydrates: 0.5g
- Protein: 1.8g
- Fat: 9.4g

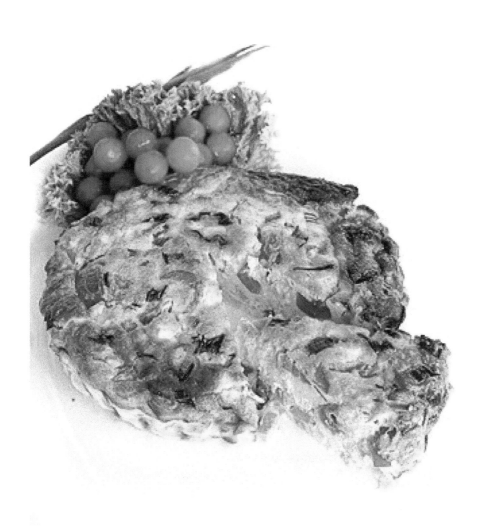

Cilantro-Lime 'n Liquid Smoke Chicken Grill

Servings per Recipe: 4

Cooking Time: 40 minutes

Ingredients:

- 1 ½ teaspoon honey /7.5ML
- 1 tablespoon lime zest /15G
- 1 teaspoon liquid smoke /5G
- 1/3 cup chopped cilantro /43G
- 1/3 cup fresh lime juice /83ML
- 2 tablespoons organic olive oil /30ML
- 3 cloves of garlic, minced
- 4 chicken breasts, halved
- Salt and pepper to taste

Instructions:

1) Put all ingredients in the bowl and allow to marinate inside the fridge for about 2 hours.
2) Preheat the air fryer to 390° F or 199°C .
3) Place the grill pan accessory within the air fryer.
4) Place the chicken on the grill and cook for 40 minutes, overturn every 10 minutes or even grill.

Nutrition information:

- Calories per serving: 571
- Carbs: 6.1g
- Protein: 60.9g
- Fat: 33.6g

Coco Milk 'n Paprika-Oregano Marinated Drumsticks

Serves: 6

Cooking Time: 30 Minutes

Ingredients:

- ½ cup almond flour /65G
- ½ cup coconut milk /125ML
- ½ teaspoon oregano /2.5G
- ½ teaspoon paprika /2.5G
- ½ teaspoon salt /2.5G
- 3 tablespoons melted butter /45ML
- 6 chicken drumsticks

Instructions:

1) Preheat the air fryer for 5 minutes
2) Soak the chicken drumsticks in coconut milk.
3) Add the almond flour, salt, paprika, and oregano to a bowl. Mix well.
4) Lightly press each side of the chicken in the almond flour mixture.
5) Place the chicken pieces inside the air fryer basket.
6) Air fry for 30 Minutes at 325° F or 163°C .
7) Shake the air fryer basket frequently for even air frying.
8) Sprinkle with melted butter once cooked.

Nutrition information:

- Calories per serving: 305
- Carbohydrates: 1.4g
- Protein: 24.1g
- Fat: 22.5g

Copycat KFC Chicken Strips

Serves: 8

Cooking Time: 20 Minutes

Ingredients:

- 1 chicken, cut into strips
- 1 egg, beaten
- 2 tablespoons almond flour /30G
- 2 tablespoons desiccated coconut /30G
- A dash of oregano
- A dash of paprika
- A dash of thyme
- Salt and pepper to taste

Instructions:

1) Soak the chicken in egg.
2) Add other ingredients to a mixing bowl and mix properly.
3) Dredge the chicken inside dry ingredients.
4) Place inside the air fryer basket.
5) Cook for 20 Minutes at 350° F or 177°C .

Nutrition information:

- Calories per serving: 100
- Carbohydrates: 0.9g
- Protein: 4.8g

- Fat: 8.6g

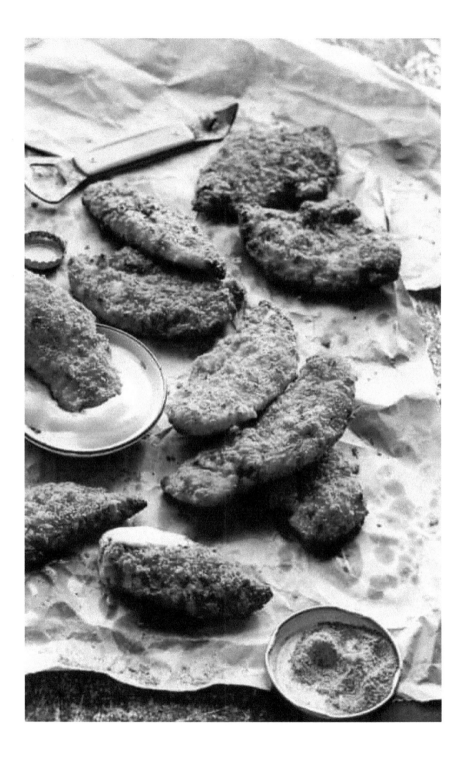

Creamy Chicken 'n Pasta Tetrazzini

Servings per Recipe: 3

Cooking Time: 30 Minutes

Ingredients:

- 1 cup chopped cooked chicken /130G
- 1/2 (10.75 ounces) can condensed cream of mushroom soup /322.5ML
- 1/2 cup chicken broth /125ML
- 1/2 cup shredded sharp Cheddar cheese /65G
- 1/4 (10 ounces) package frozen green peas /300G
- 1/4 cup grated Parmesan cheese /32.5G
- 1/4 cup minced green bell pepper 32.5G
- 1/4 cup minced onion 32.5G
- 1/4 teaspoon salt /1.25G
- 1/4 teaspoon Worcestershire sauce /1.25ML
- 1/8 teaspoon ground black pepper /0.625G
- 2 tablespoons butter /30G
- 2 tablespoons cooking sherry /30ML
- 3/4 cup sliced fresh mushrooms /98G
- 4-ounce linguine pasta, cooked following manufacturer's instructions /120G

Instructions:

1) Lightly grease baking pan of air fryer and melt butter for 2 minutes at 360° or 183°C . Stir in bell pepper, onion, and mushrooms. Cook for 5 minutes.

2) Add chicken broth and mushroom soup, mix well. Cook for 5 minutes.

3) Mix in chicken, pepper, salt, Worcestershire sauce, sherry, peas, cheddar cheese, and pasta. Sprinkle paprika and Parmesan at the top.

4) Cook for 15 minutes at 390° F or 199°C until the tops are lightly browned.

5) Serve and enjoy.

Nutrition Information:

- Calories per Serving: 494
- Carbs: 39.0g
- Protein: 28.8g
- Fat: 24.7g

Creamy Chicken 'n Rice

Servings per Recipe: 3

Cooking Time: 45 minutes

Ingredients:

- 1 (10.75 ounces) can cream of celery soup /322.5ML
- 1 (10.75 ounces) can cream of chicken soup /322.5ML
- 1 (10.75 ounces) can cream of mushroom soup /322.5ML
- 1/2 cup butter, sliced into pats /65G
- 2 cups instant white rice /260G
- 2 cups water /500ML
- 3 chicken breasts, cut into cubes
- salt and ground black pepper to taste

Instructions:

1) Grease the baking pan of the air fryer with any oil of your choice using a cooking spray.
2) Mix cream of mushroom, celery soup, chicken soup, rice, water and chicken in a pan. Mix well.
3) Season with pepper and salt. Top with butter pats.
4) Cover the pan with foil, air fry at 360° F or 183°C for 25 minutes.
5) Let it sit for 10 minutes.
6) Serve and enjoy.

Nutrition Information:

- Calories per Serving: 439
- Carbs: 36.7g
- Protein: 16.8g
- Fat: 25.0g

Creamy Chicken Breasts with crumbled Bacon

Serves: 4

Cooking Time: 25 minutes

Ingredients:

- ¼ cup essential olive oil /62.5ML
- 1 block cream cheese
- 4 chicken breasts
- 8 slices of bacon, fried and crumbled
- Salt and pepper to taste

Instructions:

1) Preheat mid-air fryer for 5 minutes.
2) Place the chicken breasts in a baking pan.
3) Add the essential olive oil and cream cheese. Season with salt and pepper to taste.
4) Place the baking dish and cook for 25 minutes at 350° F or 177°C .
5) Sprinkle crumbled bacon after air frying.

Nutrition information:

- Calories per serving: 827
- Carbohydrates: 1.7g
- Protein: 61.2g

- Fat: 67.9g

Creamy Chicken-Veggie Pasta

Servings per Recipe: 3

Cooking Time: 30 Minutes

Ingredients:

- 3 chicken tenderloins, cut into chunks
- salt and pepper to taste
- garlic powder to taste
- 1 cup frozen mixed vegetables /130G
- 1 tablespoon grated Parmesan cheese /15G
- 1 tablespoon butter, melted /15ML
- 1/2 (10.75 ounces) can condensed cream of chicken soup /322.5ML
- 1/2 (10.75 ounces) can condensed cream of mushroom soup 322.5ML
- 1/2 cup dry fusilli pasta, cooked based on manufacturer's Instructions/65G
- 1 tablespoon and 1-1/2 teaspoons essential olive oil /22.5ML
- 1-1/2 teaspoons dried minced onion /7.5G
- 1-1/2 teaspoons dried basil /7.5G
- 1-1/2 teaspoons dried parsley /7.5G
- 1/2 cup dry bread crumbs /65G

Instructions:

1) Grease the baking pan of the air fryer with oil. Add chicken and season with parsley, basil, garlic powder, pepper, salt, and minced onion. For 10 minutes, cook at 360° F or 183°C , stir halfway through cooking time.

2) Stir in mixed vegetables, mushroom soup, chicken soup, and cooked pasta. Mix well.

3) Mix well butter, Parmesan cheese, and bread crumbs in a small bowl and spread on top of casserole.

4) Cook for 20 minutes or until tops are lightly browned.

5) Serve and enjoy.

Nutrition Information:

- Calories per Serving: 399
- Carbs: 35.4g
- Protein: 19.8g
- Fat: 19.8g

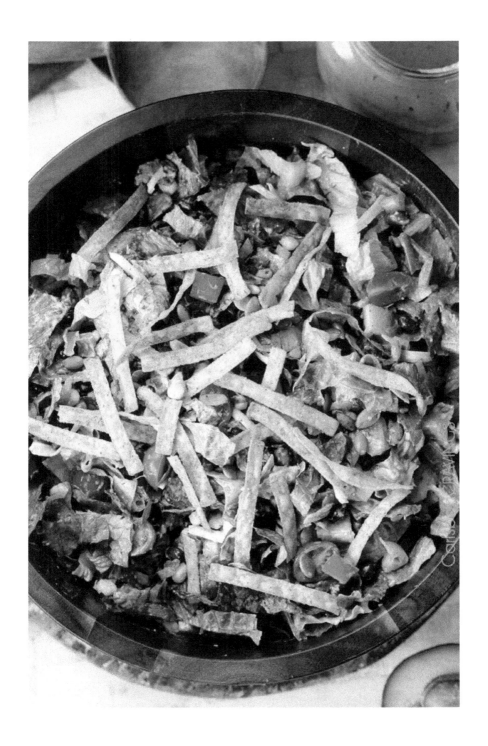

Creamy Coconut Egg 'n Mushroom Bake

Serves: 4

Cooking Time: 20 minutes

Ingredients:

- ½ cup mushrooms, chopped /65G
- 1 cup coconut cream /250ML
- 1 teaspoon onion powder /5G
- 2 tablespoons butter /30G
- 8 eggs, beaten
- Salt and pepper to taste

Instructions:

1) Preheat mid-air fryer for 5 minutes.
2) Add the eggs, butter, and coconut cream to a bowl and whisk well.
3) Pour in the baking dish, add the mushrooms and onion powder.
4) Season with salt and pepper to taste.
5) Place in the air fryer chamber and cook for 20 minutes at 310° F or 155°C .

Nutrition information:

- Calories per serving: 512
- Carbohydrates: 3.8g

- Protein: 20.8g
- Fat: 45.9g

Creamy Scrambled Eggs with Broccoli

Servings per Recipe: 2

Cooking Time: 20 Minutes

Ingredients

- 3 Eggs
- 2 tbsp Cream /30ML
- 2 tbsp Parmesan Cheese grated or cheddar cheese /30G
- Salt to taste
- Black Pepper to taste
- 1/2 cup Broccoli small florets /65G
- 1/2 cup Bell Pepper cut into small pieces /65G

Instructions:

1) Grease the baking pan of the air fryer with oil using a cooking spray. Spread broccoli florets and bell pepper on the bottom, air fry for 7 minutes at 360° F or 183°C .
2) Whisk eggs, stir in cream. Season with pepper and salt.
3) Remove the basket and pour the egg mixture over.
4) Cook for another 10 minutes.
5) Sprinkle cheese and let it sit for 3 minutes.
6) Serve and enjoy.

Nutrition Information:

- Calories per Serving: 273

- Carbs: 5.6g
- Protein: 16.1g
- Fat: 20.6g

Creamy Turkey Bake

Servings per Recipe: 5

Cooking Time: 30 Minutes

Ingredients:

- 1 can (10-3/4 ounces) condensed cream of chicken soup, undiluted /322.5ML
- 1 can (4 ounces) mushroom stems and pieces, drained /120G
- ·1 cup chopped cooked turkey or chicken
- 1 tube (12 ounces) refrigerated buttermilk biscuits, cut into 4 equal slices /360G
- 1/2 cup frozen peas /65G
- 1/4 cup 2% milk / 62.5ML
- Dash each ground cumin dried basil and thyme

Instructions:

1) Grease the baking pan of the air fryer with oil using cooking spray. Add all ingredients and mix well to combine except biscuits.
2) Top with biscuits. Cover pan with foil.
3) For 15 minutes, cook on 390° F or 199°C .
4) Remove foil and cook for 15 minutes at 330O F or until biscuits are lightly browned.
5) Serve and enjoy

Nutrition Information:

- Calories per Serving: 325
- Carbs: 38.0g
- Protein: 14.0g
- Fat: 13.0g

Crispy 'n Salted Chicken Meatballs

Serves: 6

Cooking Time: 20 Minutes

Ingredients:

- ½ cup almond flour /65G
- ¾ pound skinless boneless chicken breasts, ground /338G
- 1 ½ teaspoon herbs de Provence /7.5G
- 1 tablespoon coconut milk /15ML
- 2 eggs, beaten
- Salt and pepper to taste

Instructions:

1) Mix all ingredient in a bowl.
2) Form small balls using the hands.
3) Place inside the fridge to marinate for a couple of hours.
4) Preheat the air fryer for 5 minutes.
5) Place the chicken balls in the fryer basket.
6) Cook for 20 minutes at 325° F or 163°C .
7) Shake the fryer basket to cook evenly on every side.

Nutrition information:

- Calories per serving: 116.1
- Carbohydrates: 1.2g

- Protein: 15.9g
- Fat: 5.3g

Crispy Fried Buffalo Chicken Breasts

Serves: 4

Cooking Time: 30 Minutes

Ingredients:

- ¼ cup sugar-free hot sauce /62.5ML
- ¼ teaspoon cayenne pepper /1.25G
- ¼ teaspoon paprika 1.25G
- 1 clove of garlic, minced
- 1 cup almond flour /130G
- 1 large egg, beaten
- 1 teaspoon stevia powder /5G
- 1-pound chicken breasts, cut into thick strips /450G
- 3 tablespoons butter /45G
- Salt and pepper to taste

Instructions:

1) Preheat the air fryer for 5 minutes.
2) Season the chicken breasts with salt and pepper to taste.
3) Dip first in the beaten egg then in the flour mixture.
4) Spread the chicken breast neatly in the air fryer basket.
5) Cook for 30 minutes at 350° F or 177°C .
6) Shake the air fryer basket frequently to air fry evenly.

7) Meanwhile, to prepare the sauce, combine the remainder of the ingredients. Season the sauce with salt and pepper to taste. Set aside.

8) Once the chicken tenders are cooked, place inside a bowl with all the sauce and mix to coat.

Nutrition information:

- Calories per serving: 312
- Carbohydrates: 1.7g
- Protein: 20.4g
- Fat: 24.8g

Crispy Tender Parmesan Chicken

Serves: 2

Cooking Time: 20 Minutes

Ingredients:

- 1 tablespoon butter, melted /15ML
- 2 chicken breasts
- 2 tablespoons dairy products /30G
- 6 tablespoons almond flour /180G

Instructions:

1) Preheat mid-air fryer for 5 minutes.
2) Mix the almond flour and dairy products into a dish.
3) Sprinkle the chicken breasts with butter.
4) Dip inside the almond flour mixture.
5) Place within the fryer basket.
6) Cook for 20 minutes at 350° F or 177°C .

Nutrition information:

- Calories per serving: 712
- Carbohydrates: 1.4g
- Protein: 35.7g
- Fat: 62.6g

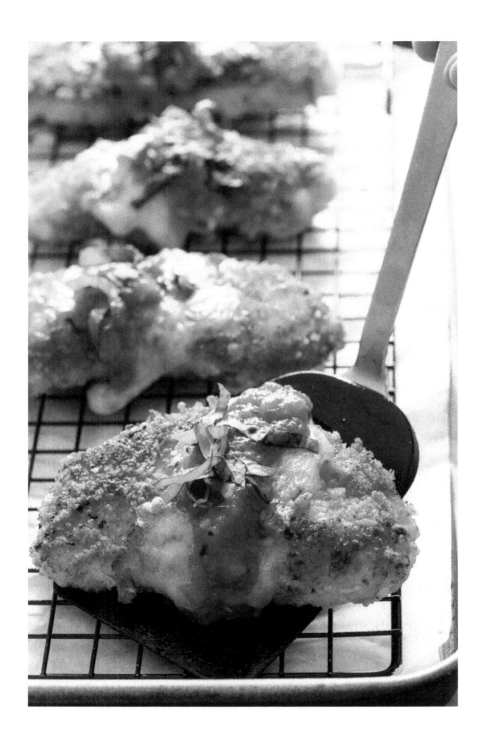

Curried Rice 'n Chicken Bake

Servings per Recipe: 3

Cooking Time: 45 minutes

Ingredients:

- 1 clove garlic, minced
- 6 ounces skinless, boneless chicken white meat halves - cut into 1-inch cubes /180G
- 1/2 cup water /125ML
- 1/2 (tall) can stewed tomatoes
- 1-1/2 teaspoons fresh lemon juice /7.5ML
- 1-1/2 teaspoons curry powder /7.5G
- 1/2 cube chicken bouillon
- 1/2 bay leaf (optional)
- 1/4 cup and 2 tablespoons quick-cooking brown rice /62.5G
- 1/4 cup raisins /32.5G
- 1/4 teaspoon ground cinnamon /1.25G
- 1/8 teaspoon salt /0.625G

Instructions:

1) Grease the baking pan of the air fryer with cooking spray.

2) While stirring add bay leaf, garlic, salt, cinnamon, bouillon, curry powder, fresh lemon juice, raisins, brown rice, stewed tomatoes, and water. For 20 minutes, cook at 360° F or 183°C . After 10 minutes of cooking time stir in chicken and mix well.

3) Cover the pan with foil.

4) Cook for 15 minutes at 390° F or 199°C , remove foil, and cook for additional 10 minutes until tops are lightly browned.

5) Serve and enjoy.

Nutrition Information:

- Calories per Serving: 247
- Carbs: 34.5g
- Protein: 22.7g
- Fat: 2.0g

Curry-Peanut Butter Rubbed Chicken

Servings per Recipe: 3

Cooking Time: 12 minutes

Ingredients:

- ½-lb boneless and skinless chicken thigh meat, cut into 2-inch chunks /225G
- 1 medium bell pepper, seeded and cut into chunks
- 1 tablespoon lime juice /15ML
- 1 tablespoon Thai curry paste /15ML
- 1 teaspoon salt /5G
- 2/3 cup coconut milk /197
- 3 tablespoons peanut butter /45G

Instructions:

1) Mix all ingredients apart from chicken and bell pepper in a bowl. Transfer half to a small bowl for basting.
2) Add chicken to the dish and mix well to coat. Marinate in the refrigerator for 3 hours.
3) Thread bell pepper and chicken pieces in skewers. Place on skewer rack in the air fryer.
4) Cook at 360° F or 183°C for 12 minutes. After 6 minutes turn over skewers and baste with sauce. If needed, cook in batches.
5) Serve and enjoy.

Nutrition Information:

- Calories per Serving: 282
- Carsbs: 10.0g
- Protein: 20.0g
- Fat: 18.0g

Dijon-Garlic Thighs

Serves: 6

Cooking Time: 25 minutes

Ingredients:

- 1 tablespoon cider vinegar /15ML
- 1 tablespoon Dijon mustard /15G
- 1-pound chicken thighs /450G
- 2 tablespoon organic olive oil /30ML
- 2 teaspoons herbs de Provence /10G
- Salt and pepper to taste

Instructions:

1) Place all ingredients in a Ziploc bag.
2) Allow to marinate inside fridge for a couple of hours.
3) Preheat air fryer for 5 minutes.
4) Place the chicken inside fryer basket.
5) Cook for 25 minutes at 350° F or 177°C .

Nutrition information:

- Calories per serving: 214
- Carbohydrates: 1.1g
- Protein: 12.7g
- Fat: 17.6g

Drunken Chicken Jerk Spiced

Servings per Recipe: 8

Cooking Time: one hour

Ingredients:

- ¾ ground cloves /
- ¾ malt vinegar
- ¾ soy sauce
- 1 ½ teaspoons ground nutmeg /7.5G
- 2 ½ teaspoons ground allspice /12.5G
- 2 tablespoons rum /30ML
- 2tablespoon salt /30G
- 4 habanero chilies
- 5 cloves of garlic, minced
- 8 pieces chicken legs

Instructions:

1) Place all Ingredients in the Ziploc bag and shake to mix. Allow to marinate inside a fridge for several hours.
2) Preheat the air fryer to 390° F or 199°C .
3) Place the grill pan accessory in the air fryer.
4) Grill the chicken for one hour and flip the chicken every 10 for even grilling.

Nutrition information:

- Calories per serving: 193
- Carbs: 1.2g
- Protein: 28.7 g
- Fat: 8.1g

Easy Chicken Fried Rice

Servings per Recipe: 3

Cooking Time: 20 Minutes

Ingredients:

- 1 cup frozen peas & carrots /130G
- 1 packed cup cooked chicken, diced
- 1 tbsp vegetable oil /15ML
- 1/2 cup onion, diced /65G
- 3 cups cold cooked white rice /390G
- 6 tbsp soy sauce /90ML

Instructions:

1) With vegetable oil lightly grease the baking pan of the air fryer. Add frozen carrots and peas.
2) Cook at 360° F or 183°C for 5 minutes.
3) Stir in the chicken and cook for an additional 5 minutes.
4) Add the remaining ingredients and mix well to combine.
5) Cook for an additional 10 minutes. Mix after 5 minutes.
6) Serve and enjoy.

Nutrition Information:

- Calories per Serving: 445
- Carbs: 59.4g
- Protein: 20.0g
- Fat: 14.1g

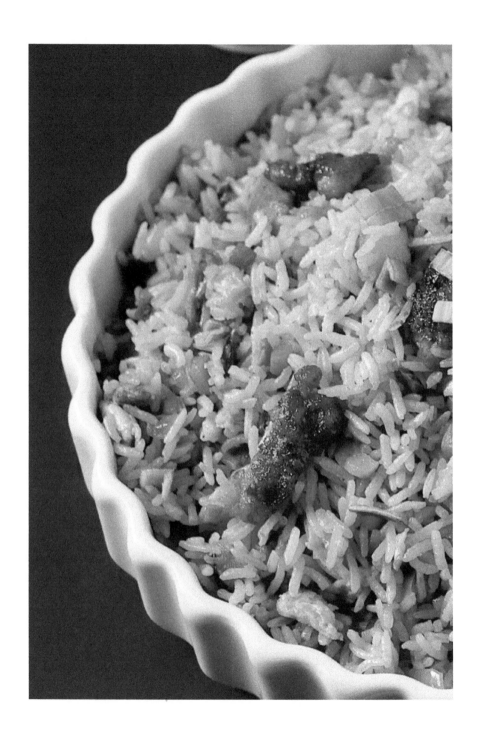

Easy Fried Chicken Southern Style

Serves: 6

Cooking Time: 30 Minutes

Ingredients:

- 1 cup coconut flour /130G
- 1 teaspoon garlic powder /5G
- 1 teaspoon paprika /5G
- 1 teaspoon pepper /5G
- 1 teaspoon salt /5G
- 5 pounds chicken leg quarters /2250G

Instructions:

1) Preheat mid-air fryer for 5 minutes.
2) Add all ingredients to a bowl and give a stir.
3) Place ingredients in the air fryer.
4) Cook for 30 minutes at 350° F or 177°C .

Nutrition information:

- Calories per serving:611
- Carbohydrates: 2.8g
- Protein: 92.7g
- Fat: 25.4g

Easy How-To Hard Boil Egg in Air Fryer

Serves: 6

Cooking Time: 15

Ingredients:

- 6 eggs

Instructions:

1) Preheat the air fryer for 5 minutes.
2) Place the eggs in the air fryer basket.
3) Cook for 15 minutes at 360° F or 183°C .
4) Remove from air fryer basket and place in cold water.

Nutrition information:

- Calories per serving: 140
- Carbohydrates: 0g
- Protein: 12g
- Fat: 10g

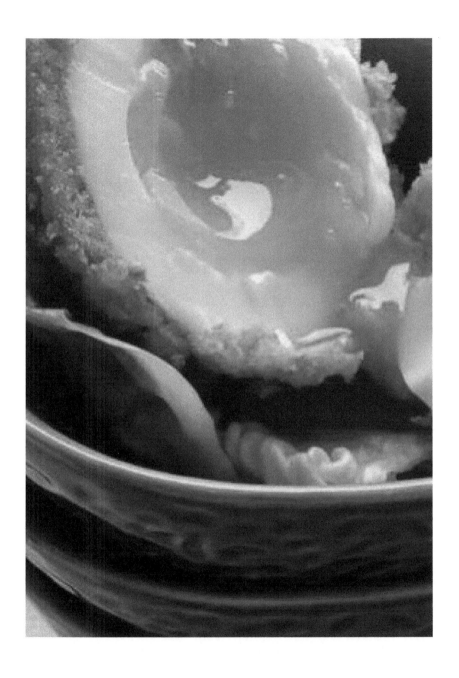

Eggs 'n Turkey Bake

Serves: 4

Cooking Time: 15 minutes

Ingredients:

- ½ teaspoon garlic powder /2.5G
- ½ teaspoon onion powder /2.5G
- 1 cup coconut milk /250ML
- 1-pound leftover turkey, shredded /450G
- 2 cups kale, chopped /260G
- 4 eggs, beaten
- Salt and pepper to taste

Instructions:

1) Preheat the air fryer for 5 minutes.
2) Add the eggs, coconut milk, garlic powder, and onion powder to a bowl and mix. Season with salt and pepper to taste.
3) Place the turkey meat and kale in the baking dish.
4) Pour in the egg mixture.
5) Place inside the air fryer.
6) Cook for 15 minutes at 350° F or 177°C .

Nutrition information:

- Calories per serving: 817

- Carbohydrates: 3.6g
- Protein: 32.9g
- Fat: 74.5g

Eggs Benedict on English Muffins

Servings per Recipe: 5

Cooking Time: 40 minutes

Ingredients:

- ½ tsp onion powder /2.5G
- 1 cup milk /250ML
- 1 stalk green onions, chopped
- 1/2 (.9 ounce) package hollandaise sauce mix
- 1/2 cup milk /125ML
- 1/2 teaspoon salt / 2.5G
- 1/4 teaspoon paprika /1.25G
- 2 tablespoons margarine /30G
- 3 English muffins, cut into 1/2-inch dice
- 4 large eggs
- 6-ounces Canadian bacon, cut into 1/2-inch dice /180G

Instructions:

1) Lightly oil the baking pan of the air fryer with cooking spray.
2) Arrange half of the bacon at bottom of the pan, Spread the dried English muffins on top. Also, spread the remaining bacon at the top.

3) Whisk the eggs, 1 cup milk, green onions, onion powder and salt well in a bowl. Pour over the English muffin mixture. Sprinkle paprika on top. Cover with foil and refrigerate overnight.

4) Preheat air fryer to 390° F or 199°C .

5) Cook in the air fryer for 25 minutes. Remove foil and continue cooking for another 15 minutes or until set.

6) Meanwhile, make the hollandaise sauce by melting margarine in a sauce pan. Mix remaining milk and hollandaise sauce in a small bowl and whisk into melted margarine. Stir continuously and simmer until thickened.

7) Serve with sauce and enjoy.

Nutrition Information:

- Calories per Serving: 282
- Carbs: 21.2g
- Protein: 17.5g
- Fat: 14.1g

Eggs, Cauliflower 'n Broccoli Brekky

Servings per Recipe: 3

Cooking Time: 20 Minutes

Ingredients:

- ½ cup milk /125ML
- ½ cup shredded Cheddar cheese /65G
- 1 cup broccoli, cut into little bits or riced /130G
- 1 cup cauliflower, riced /130G
- 1 teaspoons salt /5G
- 1/2 teaspoon ground black pepper /2.5G
- 1/2-pound hot pork sausage, diced /225G
- 3 large eggs

Instructions:

1) Oil the baking pan of the air fryer with cooking spray. And cook pork sausage for 5 minutes at 360° F or 183°C .
2) Remove basket and stir in riced cauliflower and broccoli. Cook for another 5 minutes.
3) Meanwhile, whisk well eggs, salt, pepper, and milk. Stir in cheese.
4) Remove the basket and pour in the egg mixture.
5) Cook for the next 10 minutes.
6) Serve and enjoy.

Nutrition Information:

- Calories per Serving: 434
- Carbs: 6.5g
- Protein: 27.3g
- Fat: 33.2g

French Toast with Apples 'n Raisins

Servings per Recipe: 6

Cooking Time: 40 minutes

Ingredients:

- ½ cup diced peeled apples /65G
- ½-lb loaf cinnamon raisin bread, cubed /225G
- 1 ¼ cups half-and-half cream /312.5ML
- 2 tbsp maple syrup /30ML
- 3 tbsp butter, melted /45ML
- 4 eggs
- 4-oz cream cheese, diced /120G

Instructions:

1) Lightly grease baking pan of air fryer with cooking spray.
2) Evenly spread half the bread on bottom of pan. Sprinkle evenly the cream cheese and apples. Add remaining bread ahead.
3) In a large bowl, whisk well eggs, cream, butter, and maple syrup. Pour over bread mixture.
4) Cover air fryer baking pan with plastic wrap and refrigerate for just two hours.
5) Preheat air fryer to 325° F or 163°C .
6) Cook for 40 minutes.
7) Serve while warm and enjoy.

Nutrition Information:

- Calories per Serving: 362
- Carbs: 28.3g
- Protein: 10.1g
- Fat: 23.1g

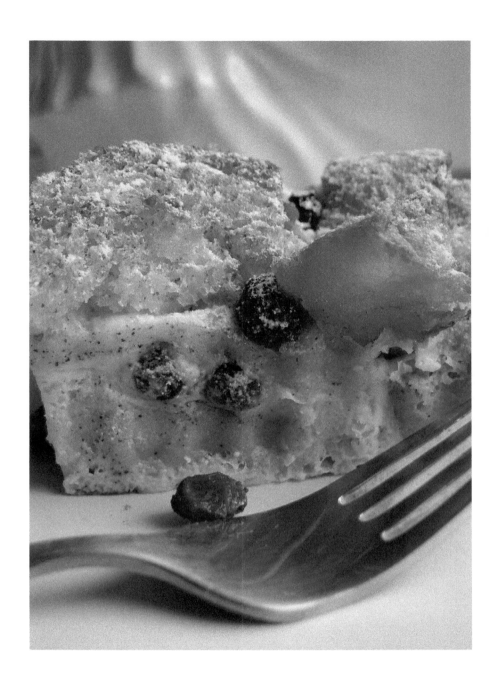

Garam Masala 'n Yogurt Marinated Chicken

Servings per Recipe: 3

Cooking Time: 40 minutes

Ingredients:

- ½ cup whole milk yogurt /125ML
- ½ teaspoon ground cumin /2.5G
- 1 ½ pounds skinless chicken thighs /675G
- 1 ½ teaspoon garam masala /7.5G
- 1 tablespoon ground coriander /15G
- 1 tablespoon smoked paprika /15G
- 1-inch ginger, peeled and chopped
- 2 tablespoons prepared mustard /30G
- 3 tablespoons fresh lime juice /45ML
- 4 cloves of garlic, minced
- 7 dried chilies, seeds removed and broken into pieces
- Salt and pepper to taste

Instructions:

1. Place all ingredients in a Ziploc bag and shake well.
2. Allow to marinate for a couple of hours in the fridge.
3. Preheat air fryer to 390° F or 199°C .
4. Place the grill pan accessory inside the air fryer.

5. Grill for about 40 minutes.

6. Flip the chicken every 10 minutes.

Nutrition information:

- Calories per serving: 589
- Carbs: 25.5g
- Protein:54.6 g
- Fat: 29.8g

Lightning Source UK Ltd.
Milton Keynes UK
UKHW020109140123
415286UK00001B/30